Foreword

An argument can be made that throughout history mankind has searched for ways to enhance brain power, while sculpting bodies resembling Greek goddesses and Roman soldiers. Anything from turning to the stars, to researching early human history, and to incorporating bionic limbs have been explored.

Yet the easiest way to unlock brain power and build six-pack abs may be to understand macro and micronutrients. Hence, *Macro and Micronutrients for Beginners*.

This book is written for anyone who values the essence of time, meaning to make the most of the 86,400 seconds in a given day. It is not meant to be a dissertation. It is instead meant to provide accurate and succinct information in an easy-to-read format. The hope is that it strikes the reader's curiosity nerve and prompts them to research in order to form their own opinions. Yes, Google is okay, but remember there is just as much false vs. right information available online today that requires veracity.

Pictures and illustrations were added in this book to take advantage of visual literacy, where just the sight of an image can enhance the communication of written words. Look for the orange color throughout the book, since this color enhances the key message.

Finally, as a subscriber to Safety First, Safety Always, consult your physician before beginning any exercise program and health-related fitness regime. The general information in this book is not intended to diagnose any medical condition or to replace your healthcare professional. Consultation with your healthcare professional to design a medically sound health-related regime is hereby advised.

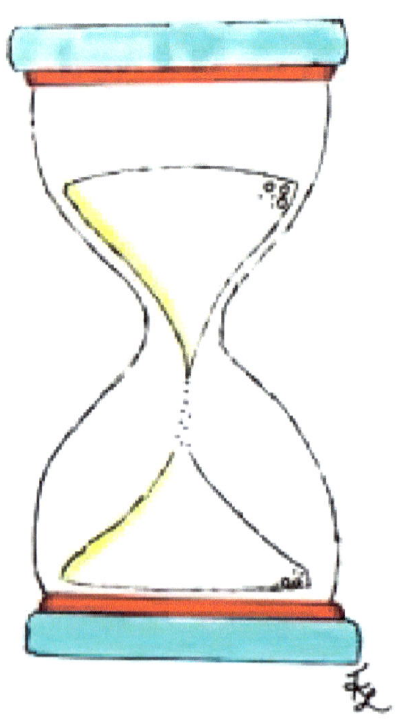

Time, Time, and Time

Time, pun intended, to be honest about how many books, journals, and news articles have you read from front to back. What about the page-turning end-user agreements or acceptance of terms and cookies that pop-up on website? Or do you rely on the chapter/book summary, cliff notes, and key takeaways rather than reading the content in its entirety?

1. Never has there been a time, pun intended again, to communicate vital information in the fastest manner possible.

2. The race for 5G (fifth generation wireless), quantum computing and understanding how particles act at the subatomic level are examples of wanting to accomplish more in shorter durations of time.

3. At a practical level, just think of the distractions going through your mind as you read this, maybe it is TikTok, maybe it is homework, or maybe it is Netflix.

4. Efficient use of time may also be a reason for communicating in alphabet soup, the OMG, SMH, TBH, ICYMI, IDK that simply speeds things up.

5. Rather than writing page after page, this book looks to provide information in an accurate and concise manner.

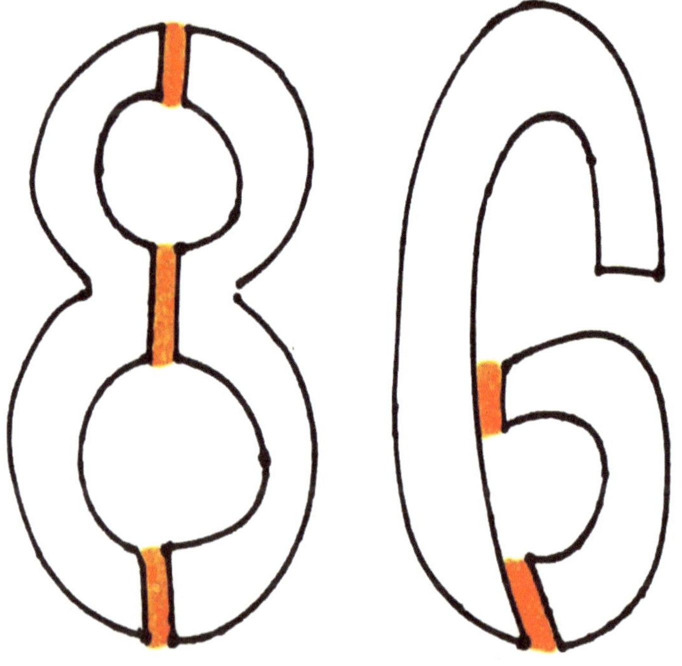

Integers Eight (8) and Six (6)

What do the integers of 8 and 6 have to do with macro and micronutrients? Why should I even care about looking at nutrients at the macro (big) and micro (small) scale when I barely have the time to cook?

1. Credit Suzana Herculano-Houzel, a neuroscientist, who found that the human brain consists of approximately 86 billion neurons.

2. In doing so, she debunked the previous number of 100 billion neurons that neuroscientist considered factual for over 50-years.

3. There are three (3) major type of neurons, sensory (e.g. touch), motor (spinal cord to muscles) and interneurons, which serve as the connection between sensory and motor (think reflexes).

4. These 86 billion neurons are at work every second of the day, which coincidentally amounts to 86,400 seconds. Hence, the integers of 8 and 6.

5. The human brain requires roughly 25%, 500 of 2000 calories, of the average daily diet to perform. Intake of sound macro and micronutrients may allow both the brain and body to perform soundly (e.g. higher IQ).

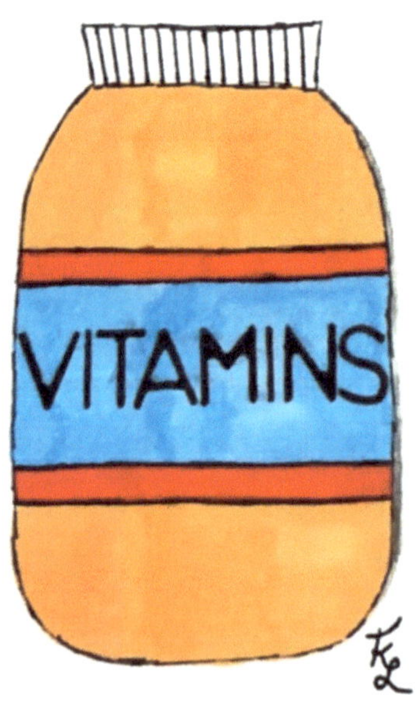
VITAMINS

Vitamins

Time to breakdown vitamins and minerals. What is the difference and similarities?

1. From a historical perspective, credit Casimir Funk, a biochemist, who was first to use the term "vital amines," which evolved to the term: Vitamins.

2. Funk broke the word down in two. Vita meant life and amine equated to meaning essential substances. Essential because the human body does not produce it, it must come from dietary intake. Important to note that Funk originally thought that every 'amine' had a nitrogen base, which we now know not to be true. This led to dropping the 'e', thus shortening the term to vitamins.

3. History aside, vitamins generally are organic substances and come in two forms: fat soluble and water soluble. Since vitamins are organic, they are susceptible to heat, light, air, and other environmental factors. So, you can destroy vitamins while cooking, which is one reason to include raw and minimally processed foods to your diet.

4. Water soluble vitamins are more easily processed in the body and any excess is literally excreted through urine. Fat soluble, on the other hand, is processed through the liver and can be stored in the body's fatty tissue. This is one reason to not over consume on fat soluble vitamins.

5. Fat soluble vitamins are vitamins A, D, E, and K. Water soluble are all of the eight (8) B complex vitamins and vitamins C. The body needs all 13 vitamins, but in different amounts and varies by age.

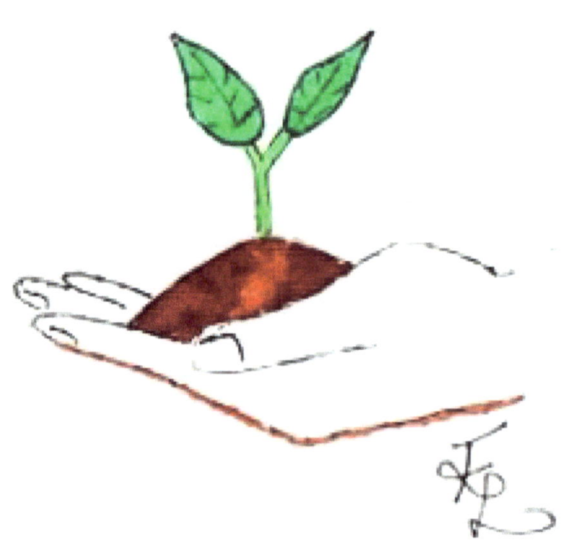

Minerals

What are minerals? What do minerals have to do we the Paleolithic age? Why is soil quality important to mineral development?

1. Unlike vitamins, minerals are inorganic elements that are present in soil and water. One way these minerals make into our food chain and food web is by way of plants.

2. The soil was rich in nutrients during the Paleolithic era, so there was not a necessity to supplement diets with multivitamin pills.

3. Soil since has been eroded of minerals, which is one reason governments fortify foods with vitamins and minerals. Stop by the milk and spices aisle next time you are in the grocery store. You may notice milk that is fortified with Vitamin D and salt contains iodine.

4. As with vitamins, minerals are broken down in two categories: major and trace. The category headers equate to quantity, where major equates large (macro) amounts and trace equates to small (micro) amounts.

5. The Harvard Health Guide on vitamins and minerals lists calcium, chloride, magnesium, phosphorus, potassium, sodium, and sulfur as major minerals. Trace minerals, on the other hand, are chromium, copper, fluoride, iodine, iron, manganese, molybdenum, selenium, and zinc. All 16 are important, but in different quantities which vary by biological sex and age of a person.

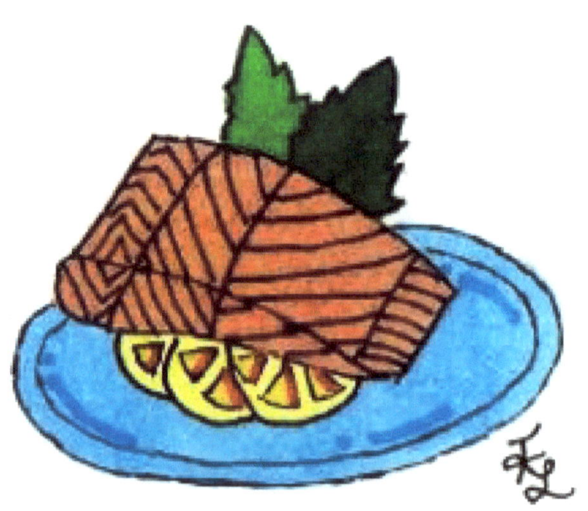

Fat

Time for yet another honest Abe moment. Do you dread upon hearing the word fat? Do yellow blob looking, excess body weight protruding images formed in the brain at just the thought of fat? If so, relax and read-on.

1. Fat is an absolute must for the brain and the body to function. Fat, at nine (9) calories of energy per gram, provides more energy than both protein and carbohydrates put together. Carbs and protein offer four (4) calories of energy per gram.

2. Dietary fat is mainly broken-down into three components: trans fat (fatty acid), saturated, and unsaturated.

3. When hydrogen is added to vegetable oil, it makes the fat more of a solid. Think margarine and vegetable shortening as examples of hydrogenated fat.

4. Saturated fat, on the other hand, is mainly found in animal products. Think of the white grisly stuff surrounding a piece of chicken or pork. Saturated fat is also found in animal by products, like in butter, whole milk, and ice cream.

5. Mono and polyunsaturated are the best source of fat for the brain and the body. Omega-3, and -6 are classified as essential fatty acids, which, like amino acids, must come from food. Oily fish happen to be the best source of omega-3, while most nuts and seeds offer the best source of omega-6

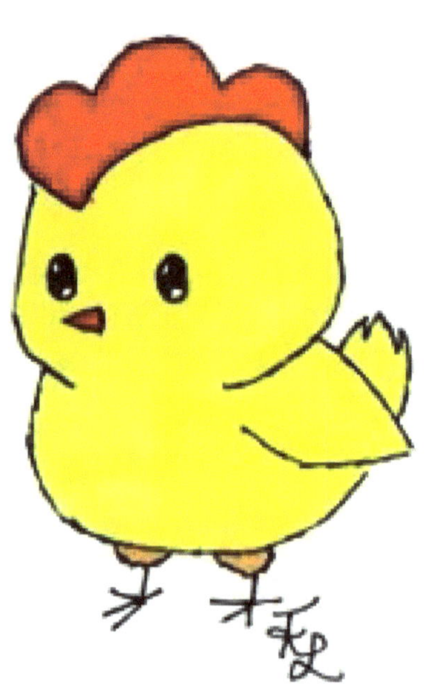

Protein

Which came first, the chicken or the chicken egg? What is the difference between complete and incomplete protein? What are essential amino acids?

1. Protein is way bigger than a macronutrient needed for building muscle. Every cell in the human body contains protein, from your hair to your nails.

2. We chug down protein shakes and wolf down chicken breasts for the nine (9) essential amino acids that are the building blocks of protein. The term essential is used because the body cannot produce these nine (9) amino acids, it must come from external sources--food.

3. Much of the protein industry uses the chicken egg as the standard for measurement, meaning does their protein stack up against the (9) amino acids found in the egg of a chicken?

4. Googling protein can be overwhelming and comical, as different sources provide different and contradictory information. Some will list beans as a complete protein, while others will suggest consuming enormous amounts, grams of protein per pound of body weight needed daily.

5. Use the Cleveland Clinic guide for a list of incomplete (e.g. legumes, nuts, seeds, vegetables, and whole grains) and complete proteins (fish, eggs, poultry, beef, pork, dairy, soy, tofu).

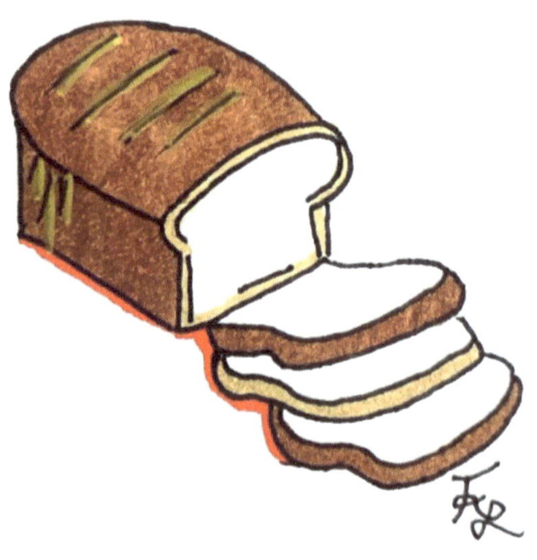

Carbohydrates

What exactly are carbohydrates? What is the difference between simple (white) and complex (brown) carbs? What is the difference between high glycemic index (GI) and low glycemic load (GL)?

1. Carbohydrates are a macronutrient and the body's preferred source for energy.

2. As the name suggests, carbohydrates are made up of three (3) elements: carbon (C), hydrogen (H), and oxygen (O). Coincidentally, carbohydrates also come in three (3) forms: sugar, starch, and fiber.

3. Glycemic index (GI) is a number, anywhere from 0 to 100, assigned to carbohydrates. GI indicates how fast or slow blood sugar will rise and can be viewed as high (70 or more), medium (56 – 69), and low (55 or less). Glucose (a type of sugar), for instance, is assigned a 100. A medium sized apple is assigned a low GI of 38 and one (1) cup of ice cream clocks in at 61.

4. Glycemic load may also be viewed as high (20 or more), medium (11 – 19), and low (10 or less). GL measures both the speed at which glucose will enter the bloodstream (GI), along with how much glucose the food contains based on the serving size. A large carrot, for instance, is assigned a GL of 2, while a snickers candy bar is assigned a GL of 35.

5. Low GI/GL foods may allow the body in regulating weight and the brain in performing efficiently, especially with the addition of essential nutrients and the removal of toxins. This is not to say that you should eliminate sugar altogether, just follow the CDC guideline of keeping the added sugar intake to 10% of daily calories.

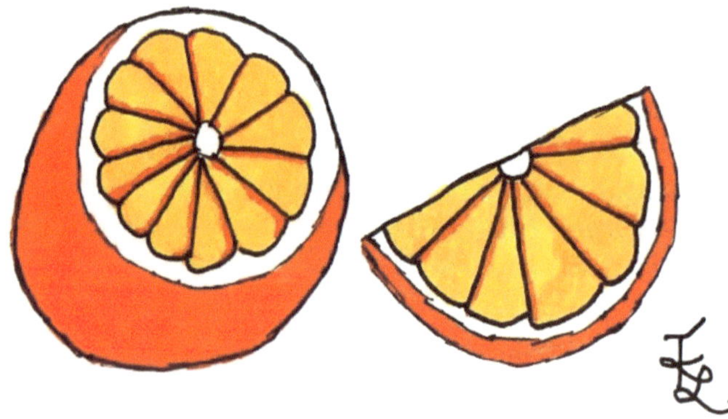

Fiber or Fibre

Quick quiz, is fiber a macro or micronutrient? What is the difference between soluble and insoluble fiber?

1. Remember, fiber is a macronutrient since it is one of the three types of carbohydrates, the other being sugar, and starch.

2. Soluble fiber just means that it dissolves in water and insoluble, as the word implies, will not dissolve in water. The human body needs both soluble and insoluble fiber.

3. The main function of soluble fiber is controlling blood sugar levels, while insoluble helps with moving food through the intestines and out the colon--think healthy bowel movements.

4. Plant cells, unlike animal cells, contain a cell wall, which the human body cannot digest. Think about an apple for a second. If peeled, the apple is easy to chew and digest. If unpeeled, the same apple takes longer to chew, and the peel goes undigested. Oranges act in the same way, the pith (white stringy stuff) is one of the healthiest parts of the orange, as it contains fiber.

5. The undigested peel is fiber, which has numerous benefits, to include satiety (feeling full), lowering blood sugar levels, and preventing diseases. One easy way to increase fiber intake is to simply leave the skin of the fruit or vegetable intact. No more peeling apples, cucumbers, potatoes, or whatever fruit and veggies that tickle your palate.

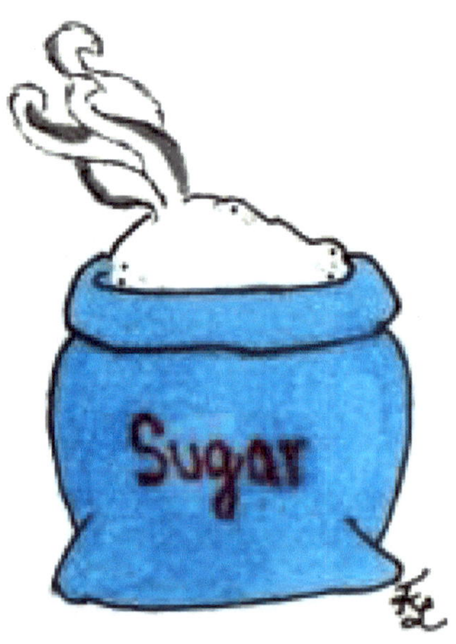
Sugar

Sugar

Does sugar cause cancer? How much sugar should be consumed in a day? Is sugar making me fat?

1. Scientist and medical experts believe that sugar by itself does not cause cancer. Consumption of excess sugar, however, is linked to an increase in fat cells. It is obesity, akin to carrying a spare around the waist, that increases the risk for cancer.

2. Sugar, regardless of the type, has four (4) calories per gram—remember, sugar is a carbohydrate. As of 2015, the World Health Organization recommends the daily caloric intake of sugar to be no more than 10%.

3. Lose the OSE, that includes dextrose, fructose, galactose, glucose, lactose, maltose, sucrose, and xylose. Generally speaking, ingredients that end with OSE, even the rose flowers, are usually a fancy way of stating sugar.

4. For a visual, check the sugar contact of your favorite bread the next time you make a sandwich. If a slice of bread contains four (4) grams of sugar, you literally are eating one packet of sugar.

5. Try substituting sugar with fruit instead. For instance, if you are part of the two billion-plus that enjoy coffee/tea, substitute sugar with a slice of an apple or orange.

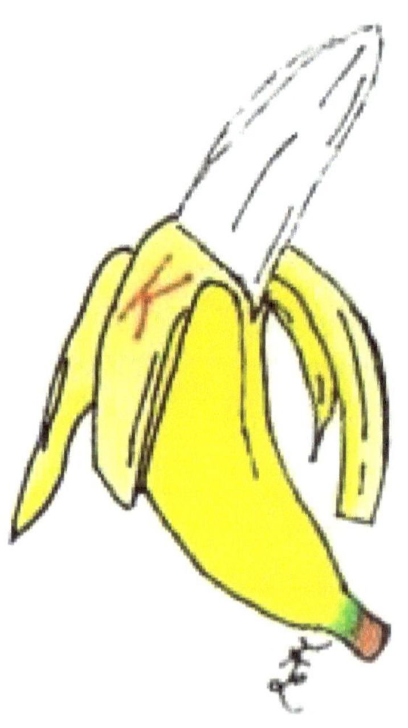

Potassium

Why is potassium referred to as an electrolyte? Can potassium help ease stress? Does the human body really conduct electricity?

1. Potassium, a mineral identified by the letter (K), is the ultimate electrolyte and de-stressor. The electrolyte moniker is used because potassium carries a small electrical charge.

2. Every cell in the body requires potassium for maintenance of normal functions. When the body stresses, like during physical exercise or medical surgery, potassium levels drop. This is one of the reasons a potassium chloride mix is given intravenously after surgeries, it helps restore the fluids and electrolytes balance.

3. Fun fact: potassium can be found in toothpaste, especially in toothpastes made for sensitivity. The potassium helps reduce the stress on the gums.

4. Try this, gather a 9V battery, a banana, and a LED or Christmas light. Use an electrical wire with alligator clips to connect both the (+) and (-) posts of the battery to the banana. Then connect the (+) and (-) legs of the LED to the banana. The led light will illuminate, proving that bananas are an electrolyte.

5. Check out the experiment on IG: 13humbles. Make sure you have adult supervision and practice safety. The battery may start getting hot if a LED light or Christmas light is not present in the banana, as the electricity will continue to run through the banana and battery.

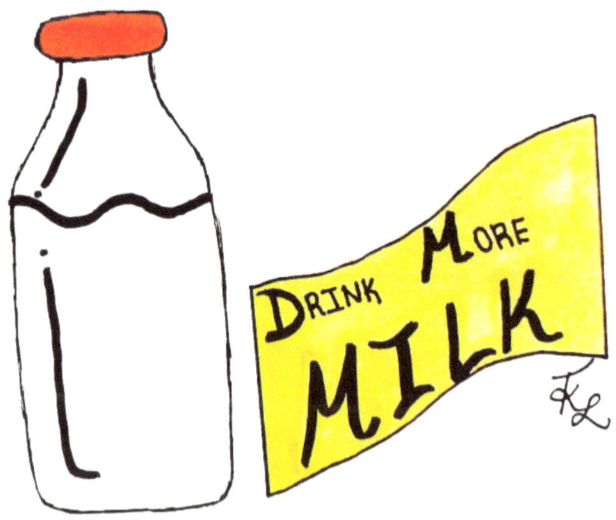
Drink More
MILK

Vitamin D

What does vitamin D have to do with sunlight? Does it really help with depression?

1. Of all the vitamins, vitamin D does not need to come from the food we eat. The human body makes its own vitamin D when exposed to sunlight.

2. The amount of sunlight, however, can be a limiting factor when it comes to vitamin D synthesis in the human body. This is also where regions of the Earth may play a factor in overall health. The closer you are to the North Pole, the more likely you are to experience an abnormal sunlight pattern.

3. For instance, Greenland, the world's largest island, experiences 4-months of light, 4-months of darkness, and 4-months of night and day. The body is unable to make vitamin D during the months of darkness due to the absence of sunlight.

4. Vitamin D comes in two (2) main forms: D2 (ergocalciferol), and D3 (cholecalciferol). D2 is produced by plants and D3 by animals. Research suggests that D3 is more important because the human body is able to absorb it better. Check out both plant and animal milk the next time you are in the dairy aisle, you may notice fortified with vitamin D on products (e.g. vitamin D milk).

5. Harvard's T.H. Chan School of Public Health cites that in laboratory studies, vitamin D has shown to reduce cancer cell growth. While the Cleveland Clinic notes that a lack of vitamin D not only leads to depression but may also cause muscle fatigue, pain, and fatigue. So, go for a walk during daytime, it will help with making vitamin D and keeping you fit.

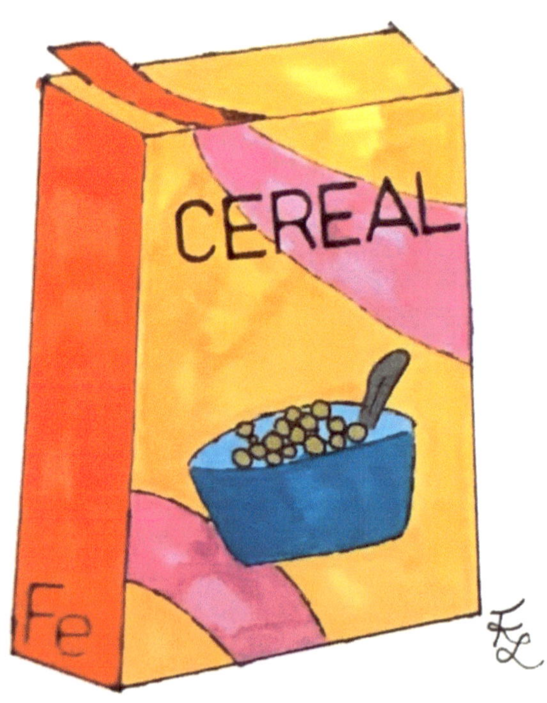

CEREAL
Fe

Iron

What is link between breakfast cereal and iron nails? Why is iron added to foods?

1. Iron, with a chemical symbol of Fe, is found throughout the universe: Stars, sun, and, of course, on Earth.

2. Iron in the human body is found in hemoglobin, which is the protein that carries oxygen through the body. Fun fact, blood gets its red color because of the iron in hemoglobin.

3. A lack of the mineral iron in the human body may lead to increased fatigue, tiredness, brain fog, trouble concentrating and a general lack of energy.

4. Observing the important role of iron in the body led food manufacturers in the early 20th century to add iron to foods like cereal. A simple experiment is carried out in elementary science classes to prove that iron is added to foods.

5. If you would like to try the experiment, crush a cup of your favorite breakfast cereal and put it in clear Ziplock bag. Add warm water to the cereal and let the mixture stand for 20 minutes or so. Then, use a refrigerator magnet and rub across the bag to see iron fillings being attracted to the magnet.

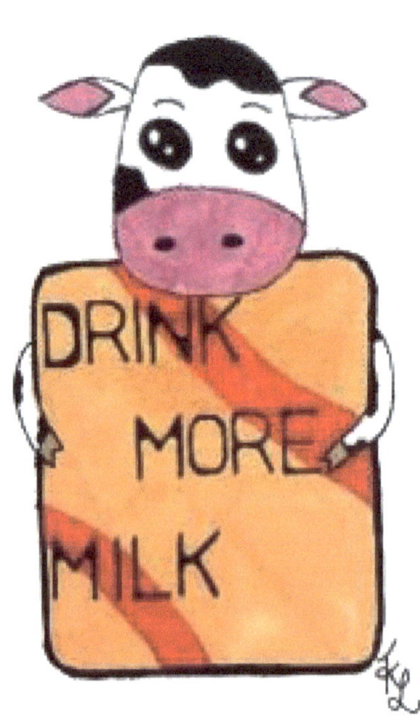
DRINK
MORE
MILK

Calcium

Do you remember the milk does your body good commercial? Or the 'Got Milk?' ad. What is the importance of milk to the body?

1. For starters, the human body does not produce (make) calcium. It must come from an external source, typically from diets containing dairy, fruits, and vegetables.

2. The other fact to remember is that, as with other minerals and vitamins, too much calcium can have negative side effects. Think of kidney stones.

3. There are two (2) types of calcium that are widely recommended: calcium carbonate and calcium citrate. Calcium carbonate has a higher concentration, meaning stronger, than calcium citrate. Fun Fact: the active ingredient in antacids, like Alka Seltzer & Tums, is calcium carbonate.

4. You may have read, heard or both that calcium prevents osteoporosis. This means that calcium keeps the bones from being too porous, containing too many holes.

5. Other than bone health, calcium is needed for proper functioning of the heart, muscles, and nerves. Keep in mind, that the body will resort to using the calcium in your bones if you are not receiving the proper amount through your diet.

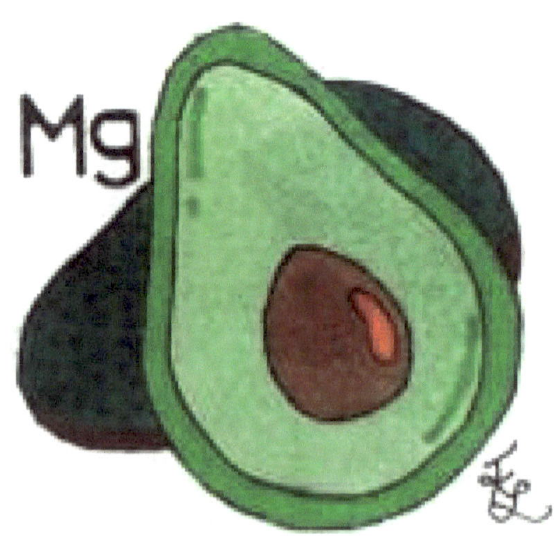
Mg

Magnesium

Do you find yourself sore and fatigued after workouts? What about being mentally drained after long days of work, study, or school? Is there something that can help with recovery of the brain and the body?

1. Magnesium is an abundant mineral found in earth, sea, plants, animals, and humans.

2. Magnesium acts like a transporter, as it helps deliver blood sugar into muscles while removing lactate. Remember lactate or lactic acid is the substance that builds up during exercise and thus causes muscle soreness.

3. There are a plethora of foods, from spinach to avocado to halibut fish, that will help meet the body's daily magnesium needs.

4. Fun fact, 33% of the Reference Daily Intake (RDI) can come from dark chocolate (70 – 85% cocoa). Eating chocolate may literally be good for you.

5. Magnesium is also critical to brain functions. In one study, scientist found that a particular compound of magnesium (L-threonate) improved learning and memory in rats. In humans, low levels of magnesium may negatively impact cognitive functions and increase the risk of depression.

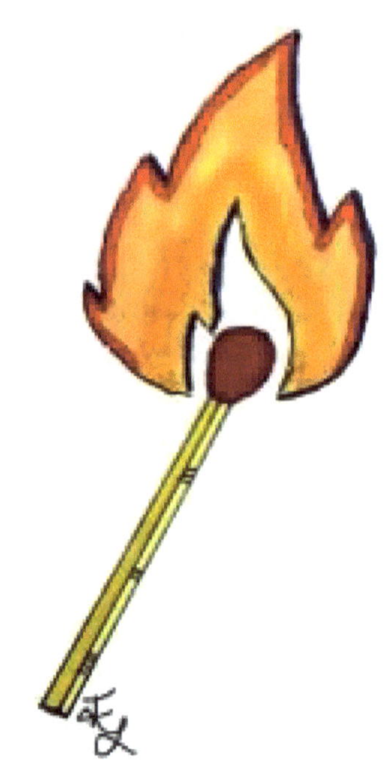

Phosphorus

Why is phosphorus sometimes referred to as the devil's element? Wait what is phosphorus anyway and why do I need it?

1. An alchemist by the name of Henning Brand discovered phosphorus by accident. He was under the impression that urine (yes, urine) and gold (yes, that gold) share the same color, so maybe there is gold in urine. Hey remember, there are no bad hypotheses.

2. Brand noticed that a glow, a light was emitted when urine was heated. He went through a few iterations of heating, then cooling, then reheating with additional urine. Different colors of light emitted with each iteration, think red and yellow glow in the dark sticks. Please, please do not try this at home!

3. Naturally, he named the substance Phosphorus, Greek for light bearer. This glow and the fact that it was the 13th element discovered is why some refer to it as the "devil's element."

4. Henning did not necessarily know that he discovered one of the most essential elements of life. Phosphorus is needed for healthy bones, teeth, nerve functions and is vital to cellular growth and development since it is also a component of DNA and RNA.

5. Fun fact: match sticks and match boxes are a great example of phosphorus glowing and volatile nature. The striking side of the match box contains red phosphorus, while the head of the matchstick contains white phosphorus. When struck, the friction between the two surfaces produces fire. One other note, roughly 1% of a person's body weight may be attributed to phosphorus.

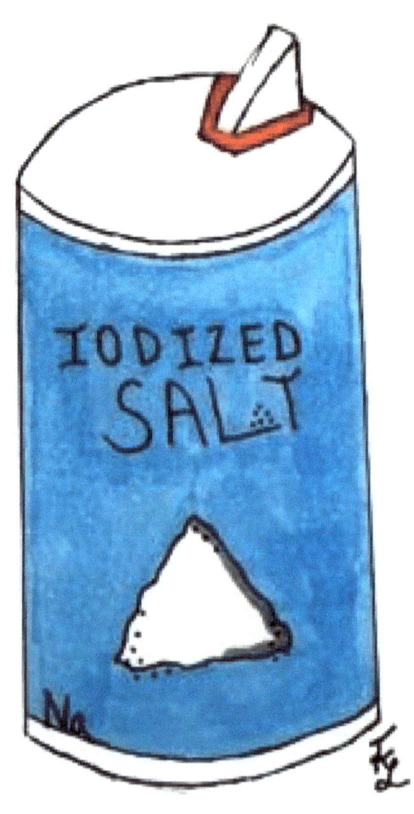
IODIZED
SALT
Na

Iodized Salt

Wait, there is iodine in my salt? Why?

1. The value of salt is unlike any of the other minerals. Salt can be found in religious texts, in shaping of cultures, in economical use, in medicine, and in general development of civilizations across the world. It predates recorded history.

2. In recorded history, the Roman Empire used salt to pay their soldiers. The word salt eventually transitioned to salary. Wars were even won and lost due to salt. Historians believe that thousands of Napoleon's soldiers died during the retreat from Moscow because salt was unavailable. Salt was used to heal wounds.

3. Fast forward to early 20th century for understanding why salt is fortified with iodine. Iodine can prevent the development of goiters, which is an enlargement of the thyroid gland. Google goiters and you are likely to see images of people with large lumps in their neck.

4. Salt, referred to as sodium chloride by chemists, helps maintain nerve functions and fluid levels. Too much salt, however, causes hypertension or high blood pressure.

5. Excess salt can harden the arteries, which taxes the heart since it has to work harder to circulate blood around the body. Fun fact, salt and pepper are regarded as a couple, so make sure to pass them together at the dining table.

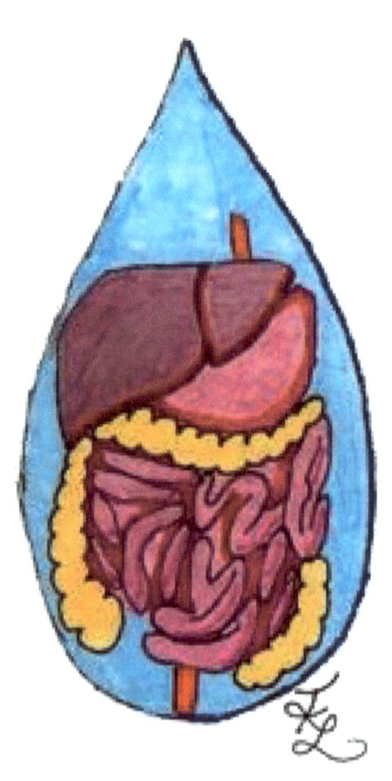

Water, Water, and Water

What is the connection between indoor plumbing and the human digestive system? Why does every sensible medical and plumbing professional call for water?

1. Water is the first, the in-between, and the last vital nutrient you may want to include in your everyday diet.

2. The human body, skin, bones, muscle, and the brain are porous, meaning that their holes of the macro, micro and nano sizes.

3. The human digestive system closely resembles indoor plumbing, where the stomach/bladder acts like the toilet bowl, the intestines act like plumbing lines, and the colon acts like a flush. Coincidently, both plumbing and the body rely on gravity to aid with flushing toxins.

4. If there is not enough water and pressure, then sentiments, smells, and streaks may be found in the toilet, as well as within the digestive system.

5. Nasty visuals aside, you want enough water to transport nutrients, while removing the toxins the first go-around.

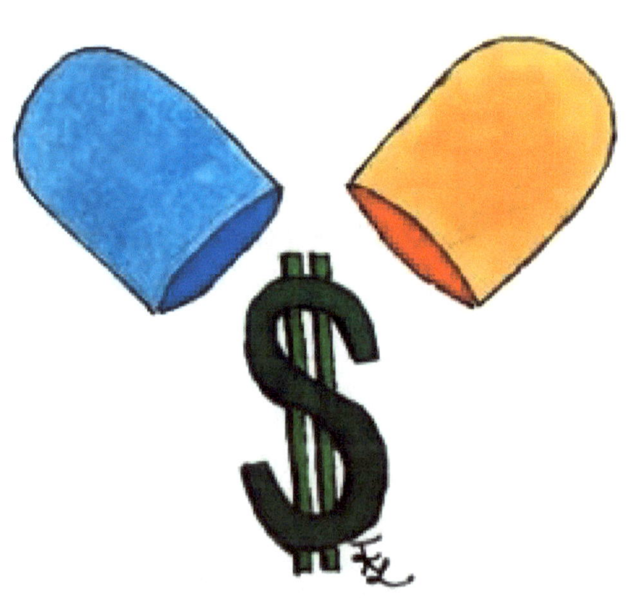

Dollars & Sense

Okay, so do multivitamins work? Is it worth the money? Are all multivitamins the same? And why do gummie vitamins taste better than tablets?

1. Zion Market Research estimated the global dietary supplements market to be around $132.8 billion in 2016. This number increases to $220.3 billion by 2022. Statista forecasts that the average revenue per person will amount to $2.62 in 2020, meaning each person will spend $2.62 on multivitamins and minerals.

2. To be clear, the supplement market, which includes botanicals, vitamins, minerals, amino acids, & enzymes, began in the 1940s and stemmed from meeting nutrition needs for soldiers during WWII. Safe to say, this market is not going anywhere.

3. All multivitamins are definitely not the same. Some tablets, for instance, may contain binders and fillers that the body is unable to breakdown. Think of binders as a type of glue used to keeping the powder in tablet form, which may prevent the body from absorbing the nutrients. In that case, you literally paid for nothing. Enter mouth, exit colon.

4. The National Institute of Health Office of Dietary Supplements is a good place to start, refer to the Vitamin and Mineral Supplement Fact Sheets.

5. Ultimately, research supports both using supplements and& sticking to food for meeting individual multivitamin and mineral needs. Eating a well-balanced diet, however, will not only save you money but promises to be the best method to meeting the recommended dietary intakes.

About the Author

I have failed so many times, both academically and in life, that I decided to subscribe to the 5Fs of life: Faith, Family, Fitness, Fellowship, and Fun. I do not possess any combination of the 26 letters in English for expressing my gratitude for the countless people who have shaped my perspectives.

I would, however, like to specifically thank my students, from kinder to adults, who have motivated me in more ways than I can count. Their teachings have left me with an unyielding motivation for wanting to learn more of how the body and brain work.

Furthermore, I would like to thank Fiza, the illustrator and aspiring fashion designer, whose artwork should convey messages faster than processing of words. Last, but not least, a special mention of my editor extraordinaire(s), Ann, Ericka, and Remelia. This book would not have been possible without them, they are an absolute blessing!

Chetan recently earned his doctorate in education, with his dissertation on understanding the impact of obesity on academic performance in elementary students. He is also a 21-year Air Force veteran (retired Chief Master Sergeant), a public-school and university science, technology, engineering, and mathematics teacher, a certified personal trainer, and, most importantly, a lifelong student.

Connect with the author on T: @13humbles, and IG: 13humbles.

www.ingramcontent.com/pod-product-compliance
Lightning Source LLC
Chambersburg PA
CBHW040315240726
48664CB00006B/1495